Avoiding Common Pitfalls in Medical Writing

An Editor's Advice

Deanna Erin Conners, MS, PhD

MILNE OPEN TEXTBOOKS
GENESEO

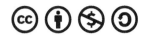
ISBN: 978-1-956862-08-9

Published by Milne Open Textbooks, Milne Library
State University of New York at Geneseo,
Geneseo, NY 14454

This e-book is dedicated to my parents,
David and Rosemary Conners,
who always nurtured my curiosity and supported my love of
the sciences.

Contents

The Publication Process

Live Audiences

Introduction

Scientific literature offers an important window into the way the world works, and being able to contribute to this body of knowledge is a privilege. In an ideal world, all scientific papers would start out as clear, concise, and compelling descriptions of scientific research. However, early-career researchers are still learning how to write well, and mid- and late-career researchers are busy people—editors work to help bridge this gap in quality between first drafts and final masterpieces.

The following pages contain editorial advice for avoiding common mistakes and addressing other problematic issues scientists and others encounter when writing in the field of biomedicine. This advice, in the form of brief (1–3 page) educational factsheets, was compiled over the first two years of running a scientific editing program at Roswell Park Comprehensive Cancer Center in Buffalo, NY.[1] The editing program shares these factsheets with our faculty clients and trainees through educational efforts to improve writing. Now, I am pleased to offer this advice in an open format where the content will be discoverable, accessible, and usable by a wider audience. Suggested uses are with students in the classroom, postgraduate trainees in mentorship programs, new editors during professional development activities, and faculty receiving editing support from faculty development and research development programs.

Each factsheet was designed to provide a quick overview of a timely editorial topic written in a friendly, supportive tone, with much of the content based on common knowledge in the field of scientific editing. A few further readings and resources are offered within particular factsheets to allow readers to take a deeper dive into the topic at hand. This e-book concludes with a Recommended Further Readings and Resources section, which details more comprehensive and authoritative resources on academic scientific writing that all writers and editors should keep close by when working on a project. Lastly, I encourage you to seek additional advice from the many great blogs on scientific writing produced by diverse scientific editors (too many to attempt to list in this e-book). There are surely other gems of advice waiting to be discovered.

---

1. Conners, D.E., Brooks, J.L., Epstein, J.G., & Gollnick, S.O. (2023). Ten Lessons Learned from Starting a New Scientific Editing Program at a Comprehensive Cancer Center. *Science Editor*, 46, 86–89. https://doi.org/10.36591/SE-D-4603-01

Humbly, I now offer you the following words of advice I have accumulated over my multiple years as a scientific editor. On your journey, may your publication successes be many and your rejections few.

WRITING AND STYLE BASICS

1 | Three Types of Editing: Proofreading, Copy Editing, and Content Editing

Key Point

Editing will benefit your writing, regardless of whether you are a seasoned scientist with many high-impact publications or an early-career investigator cranking out your first grant proposals.

Best Practices

The three main types of editing performed by scientific editors, and at times by the authors/co-authors themselves or supportive colleagues, are proofreading, copy editing, and content editing. Learning about these different types of editing services and when they are appropriate to use will help you to become more efficient at producing high-quality grant proposals and manuscripts.

Proofreading

In modern parlance, proofreading refers to skimming a polished paper or proposal to look for inadvertent errors in grammar, punctuation, spelling, and formatting that were missed during earlier review steps. It is the quickest type of editing. Oftentimes, authors perform the final reading because they are most familiar with the content. Because it is hard to edit your own work, check the proof with fresh eyes (that is, after taking a break from writing) and in a different format, such as a PDF versus Microsoft Word file or a print out. Reading the text aloud is also very helpful for catching proofreading errors.

Copy Editing

Copy editing takes more time than proofreading but is still relatively quick. This work involves both the above corrections for the mechanics (grammar and so forth) and also minor to moderate improvements in style or clarity. For example, topic sentences may be recommended to aid in the flow of logic, acronyms, or technological concepts may be defined or explained in more detail, and headings may be changed to achieve a parallel structure. All academic documents stand to benefit from a good copy edit by someone with fresh eyes who is also familiar with scientific style and formatting conventions. Hence, do not hesitate to ask for editing support—even the best writers commonly employ an editor. Typically, that person is an editor at a journal, an editor affiliated with either an academic organization or editing company, or a senior colleague.

Content Editing

Content editing, also called substantive editing, is the most time consuming of the three types of editing. In conjunction with the above copy editing work, a content editor may make extensive changes to improve clarity and logic and better highlight the significance and novelty. Furthermore, additional text and keywords may be recommended (or organizational changes made) to demonstrate the alignment with a journal's scope or funder's priorities. Conversely, deletions may be recommended if the text is redundant or tangential. Content editing is typically carried out by an experienced scientific editor.

Whatever type of editing support you seek, view the experience as an educational opportunity to improve your writing skills. If you pay careful attention to the changes that were made, you will be more likely to avoid the same pitfalls in future writing projects. A brief conversation with your editor beforehand about what type of editing is being sought or will be provided can be beneficial for professional collaborations. In addition, if there are questions after the edits are returned, a conversation with the editor may be useful to clarify the problems identified and determine the appropriate solutions.

2 | When to Use the Past and Present Tense of Verbs

> *Key Point*
>
> Use past tense when referring to your own methods and results in a scientific document. Use present tense when referring to well known facts or previously published research that is now accepted as factual.

Best Practices

Scientific papers and proposals contain a mixture of verb tenses, and it can be challenging to know which tense to use. The tense of a verb is used to distinguish among past, present, or future times. In scientific documents, the past tense is used to discuss actions that occurred in the past. Hence, the methods and results sections are written primarily in the past tense. For example, "fluorescence *was* measured on a spectrofluorometer," "the results *showed* that treatment A worked better than treatment B."

The present tense is used when referring to well known facts or previously published research that is now widely considered to be factual. For example, "cancer *is* one of leading causes of death in the United States," "a previous study demonstrated that immune checkpoint inhibitors *are* useful for treating advanced melanoma." The present tense is used in these situations because the fact itself is not expected to change over time. Therefore, the present tense is used frequently in the introduction section of a paper, and it also may be used in the discussion. Additionally, the present tense is used when referring directly to a table or figure, for example, "Figure 1 *shows* that the tumors decreased in size over the course of three weeks."

These general guidelines will apply to most scientific writing projects. However, check the journal's author guidelines for any specific tense advice and follow it. While it is rare, a few journals prefer authors use present tense for their own results. The author guidelines should always be given preference if there is any discrepancy as to what style should be used in a scientific paper.

3 | Break up Looooong Sentences

> **Key Point**
>
> Break up long sentences to improve the readability of your paper.

Best Practices

Long sentences can be difficult to read, especially when the content is technical or complex. The readability of your manuscript or grant proposal will be enhanced immensely if lengthy blocks of text are broken up into smaller fragments that are easier for readers to digest. Several grammatical tools are available for breaking up the sentence structure, including periods, semicolons, and em dashes.

The simplest approach is to use a period to separate independent clauses when the sentence becomes long and unwieldy. While there is no straightforward rule to how long a sentence should be—variation in sentence length can actually make writing more interesting—sentences that are longer than 20–25 words can pose challenges to reader comprehension. Hence, scrutinize sentences that are longer than two or three lines to determine if these can be made shorter.

Use a semicolon to break up a rambling sentence when it makes sense to retain some sort of connection between the independent clauses. In the example below, Charles Darwin used a semicolon in the last sentence of *On the Origin of Species*,[1] which was written in 1859:

> *There is grandeur in this view of life, with its several powers, having been originally breathed into a few forms or into one; and that, whilst this planet has gone cycling on according to the fixed law of gravity, from so simple a beginning endless forms most beautiful and most wonderful have been, and are being, evolved.*

Finally, use an em dash to interject ideas and information that deserve more emphasis than a parenthetical phrase or fragment set off by commas—this type of dash is especially helpful when the interjected material contains commas. Em dashes are longer than hyphens and en dashes, and these symbols can be inserted by using the Insert > Symbol function in Microsoft Word. As shown below, Douglas Hanahan and Robert Weinberg artfully used em dashes in their seminal paper titled "Hallmarks of Cancer: The Next Generation" in *Cell*:[2]

> *The six hallmarks of cancer—distinctive and complementary capabilities that enable tumor growth and metastatic dissemination—continue to provide a solid foundation for understanding the biology of cancer.*

Readers will benefit from your efforts to simplify the text by breaking up long, unwieldy sentences.[3]

---

1. Darwin, C. & Kebler, L. (1859). On the origin of species by means of natural selection, or, The preservation of favoured races in the struggle for life. London: J. Murray. [Pdf] Retrieved from the Library of Congress. https://www.loc.gov/item/06017473/

2. Hanahan, D. & Weinberg, R.A. (2011). Hallmarks of Cancer: The Next Generation. *Cell*, 144, 646–647. https://doi.org/10.1016/j.cell.2011.02.013

3. This content would be useful for a training exercise in which participants are asked for their ideas on how to apply the above three tools to break up a long, rambling sentence that might appear in a scientific paper or grant proposal.

4 | Unusual Places Where You Need to Use a Comma

Key Point

Commas are punctuation marks that indicate a pause in a sentence and help make the text easy to understand.

Best Practices

Many people know that you need to routinely use a comma in certain places including (1) before a conjunction (and, but, or, nor, for, yet, so) to separate two independent clauses in a sentence ("proteins were quantified by Western blots, and DNA was extracted for Sanger sequencing"), (2) after introductory phrases such as "however" and "lastly", and (3) to set off phrases or clauses that are not essential to the meaning of a sentence, both at the beginning and end of the phrase. Moreover, many people have already formed an opinion about serial commas, also known as Oxford commas, which are the commas inserted before the last item in a list of three or more items. Some people use these in all lists, whereas others do not (our editing program recommends the consistent use of the serial comma). Always use a serial comma when necessary for clarity (there is ambiguity in this sentence, "The scientists she admires most include her postdoctoral mentors, Elizabeth Blackburn and Marian Koshland"; the serial comma makes clear the author is referring to more than two people, "The scientists she admires most include her postdoctoral mentors, Elizabeth Blackburn, and Marian Koshland").

Here are a few unusual places where the appropriate insertion of a comma will show off your impeccable writing style:

1. After the year in a date with a month, day, and year. For example, "The National Cancer Act signed into law on December 31, 1971,[1] provided the necessary framework for today's cancer center program, data collection efforts through SEER (Surveillance, Epidemiology, and End Results Program), and the National Clinical Trials Network." No commas are needed when only the month and year are given or when writing the date in the British English style or international date format (31 December 1971).

2. After a geographic location with a city and state. For example, "Buffalo, New York, won a Golden Snow Globe award for being the snowiest city in the United States with over 100,000 residents during the winter of 2018–2019."[2]

3. Before and after a degree. For example, "Gerty Theresa Cori, née Radnitz, MD, was the first woman to win the Nobel Prize in Physiology or Medicine[3] for her research on carbohydrate metabolism, much of which was carried out at Roswell Park (then the State Institute for the Study of Malignant Diseases) during the 1920s."

4. In between coordinating adjectives (thoughtful, intelligent students) but not non-coordinate adjectives (bright green dye). Coordinate adjectives can be identified by the fact that you can reverse their order or write "and" in between them without changing the meaning.

5. After and around interjections. For example, "Indeed, the results supported the hypothesis that the protein is a viable target for anticancer therapies."

Above are common places where people often get tripped up in their academic writing. For a more comprehensive refresher on commas, visit Purdue OWL's (Online Writing Lab) website on Extended Rules for Using Commas.[4]

1. Alam, N. (2021, December 10). *Impact of 1971's National Cancer Act marked*. NIH Record. https://nihrecord.nih.gov/2021/12/10/impact-1971-s-national-cancer-act-marked

2. *2018 – 2019 US City Snowfall Totals | Golden Snow Globe National Snow Contest Snowiest US City Pop 100,000+*. (n.d.). https://goldensnowglobe.com/all-past-snow-seasons-winners/2018-2019-us-city-snowfall-totals/

3. The Nobel Prize. (2024, October 17). *Gerty Cori – Biographical*. https://www.nobelprize.org/prizes/medicine/1947/cori-gt/biographical/#content

4. Purdue University. (n.d.). *Extended rules for Using commas*. Purdue Online Writing Lab. https://owl.purdue.edu/owl/general_writing/punctuation/commas/extended_rules_for_commas.html

5 | How to Avoid Comma Splices

Best Practices

Scientific papers contain numerous clauses, both independent and dependent, which are joined by various punctuation marks and connecting words. Independent clauses are those that form a complete sentence with a subject and verb. The examples below illustrate the incorrect and correct ways that independent clauses can be connected by comma splices, periods, semicolons, and comma–conjunction combinations:

- INCORRECT: Several tumors decreased in size, a few tumors showed no change.
- CORRECT: Several tumors decreased in size. A few tumors showed no change.
- CORRECT: Several tumors decreased in size; a few tumors showed no change.
- CORRECT: Several tumors decreased in size, but a few tumors showed no change.

While comma splices are fairly common in poetry and fiction—one of the most famous splices by Charles Dickens reads "It was the best of times, it was the worst of times ..."—use of this grammatical technique should be avoided in scientific writing. In scientific writing, the best approach is to maintain a formal tone with strict adherence to grammatical conventions.

6 | How to Stop Dangling Your Participles

> *Key Point*
>
> Position a participle, which often takes the form of a verb ending in -ing, next to the noun that it modifies. When the participle is placed too far away from its subject or lacks a subject, the result is a grammatical error known as a dangling participle.

Best Practices

A participle is a verbal form that serves as an adjective.[1] Present participles end in -ing (e.g., showing, writing), whereas past participles have various endings, such as -ed, -t, -n (e.g., showed, written).

A dangling participle is a grammatical error in which the participle is not clearly related to the noun (or noun phrase) that it is modifying. This can occur when the participle is positioned next to the wrong noun (too far away from the intended one) or when there is no noun for it to modify. This is a very common error in scientific documents, and examples are given below.

This sentence contains a misplaced participle phrase: "Having experience with CRISPR technologies, the proposed research will benefit from the involvement of Dr. Noteworthy."

---

1. Merriam-Webster. (n.d.). Participle. In *Merriam-Webster.com dictionary*. Retrieved from https://www.merriam-webster.com/dictionary/participle

The doctor, not the proposed research, possesses the experience. One way to correct this dangle is to rearrange the text, "Dr. Noteworthy, having experience with CRISPR technologies, will be a valuable member of the proposed research team." Or you can lose the participle all together, "The proposed research will benefit from the involvement of Dr. Noteworthy, who has experience with CRISPR technology."

The following sentence is missing a noun for the participle using: "Mice were photographed using a camera as they explored different features of the new habitat." What talented mice! The simplest fix here is to add the subject to the participle phrase as follows: "We used a camera to photograph the mice as they explored ..."

A quick (but not always best[2]) fix for dangling forms of "using" is to replace or supplement the term with a preposition, such as "with," "by means of," or "by using."

While many people can figure out the meaning of a sentence with a dangling participle, the interpretation process takes time and detracts from the writing quality. Avoid dangling participles.

2. Shearson Editorial Services. (2011, February 15). *A lost cause? Dangling "using."* https://www.shearsoneditorial.com/2011/02/a-lost-cause/

SPECIALIZED STYLE CONCERNS

7 | How to Use and Format Acronyms

Key Point

Define all acronyms upon first use in an abstract and again in the main text of a paper. Once an acronym has been defined, use it thereafter.

Best Practices

Acronyms help us to communicate scientific content quickly. However, the use of too many acronyms or the improper use of acronyms can hamper reader comprehension. Best practices for using acronyms in papers include the following.

Define the acronym at its initial point of use in the abstract and again in the main text.

Once an acronym has been defined in the main text, use it thereafter (though repeat definitions are acceptable in the conclusions of a long paper and figure and table captions).

Avoid the use of acronyms in titles (with the rare exception of a lengthy gene name, most title words should be spelled in full to make the content readable for a broad audience).

Do not use an acronym if the phrase is used rarely—though it may be appropriate to use such an acronym for organization names and methodological names that are best known by their acronyms, e.g., NIH, HPLC.

Use acronyms judiciously while balancing the competing needs for brevity and clarity for non-technical readers.

If your paper contains numerous acronyms, consider creating a list of abbreviations to be published along with the text if space allows, as this will aid in reader comprehension.

Typically, the acronym is defined in full before the parentheses and the acronym itself is given within the parentheses. However, if the definition is too disruptive to the flow of the text (e.g., a gene name), you may write the acronym first and place the full definition in parentheses—apply this technique sparingly. Similarly, reverse order may be appropriate for organizational names if the entity is better known by its acronym.

While some journals do allow the use of a few common acronyms without definition, for example, DNA and RNA, it is usually best to define the term if there is any doubt as to what is acceptable for a particular journal.

The above advice applies to grant proposals too. In particular, define all acronyms at their point of first use in each section of a grant proposal because reviewers may skip to different sections. Introductory sections (Summary, Project Narrative, Specific Aims) must always be written as stand-alone documents, i.e., be understood without having to refer to other sections.

8 | How to Express Numbers in Scientific Documents

Key Point

In general, all numbers with a unit or those that are 10 or greater should be written as numerals. Style guides vary as to whether one should spell out cardinal numbers less than 10 or write these as numerals; the former style is preferred in business documents, while the latter style is preferred in technical documents. Ordinal numbers (ranks) from first to ninth should always be spelled out.

Best Practices

Scientific documents are full of numbers. Many of these numbers are associated with units, whereas others are not. When writing about a number with a unit, for example, 70 kg, 1 mL, and 2 h, use a numeral. If the number is not associated with a unit, use numerals for numbers that are 10 or greater and consult the author instructions for the best approach to use for cardinal numbers less than 10 (five mice or 5 mice). The latest guidance from the American Medical Association (AMA) and Council of Science Editors (CSE) states that authors should largely use numerals for cardinal numbers less than 10 in scientific documents (occasionally, zero or one may need to be written out for clarity), but not all journals have adopted this new convention.

There are two important exceptions to the above general rule: lists and multiplication terms. Specifically, if you have a list of numbers in which one of the numbers is 10 or greater, then use numerals for all of the numbers, for example, "a total of 8, 12, and 5 replicates were used for experiments A, B, and C, respectively." Similarly, if you are writing about a multiplication term, then always use a number, for example, 2 times, 4 fold.

In the rare instance that a sentence begins with a number, spell out the number regardless of whether it has a unit or not. Oftentimes, for brevity, you can just reword or rearrange the text. Examples of each approach are as follows:

- One milliliter of solution A was added to the beaker.
- Next, 1 mL of solution A was added to the beaker.

Another rare situation is when two numbers are written next to each other in a series. In these cases, it is acceptable to spell out one number and use a numeral for the other regardless of the above general rule. For example, one could write "twelve 3 cm tumors" for clarity. Hyphens are also helpful to employ in such situations (two 3-day conferences).

Lastly, spell out and hyphenate fractions that appear in the text. For example, "approximately two-thirds of the population were not aware that alcohol consumption is a risk factor for the development of cancer."[1]

Further readings and resources

- Livingstone, E.H. Numbers and Percentages, Chapter 18. In: *AMA Manual of Style: A Guide for Authors and Editors*, 11th Edition. American Medical Association (AMA), Oxford University Press, 2020.
- Lang, T.A., Ancker, J.S., and Lambert, R. (eds.) Numbers, Units, Mathematical Expressions, and Statistics, Chapter 12. In: *The CSE Manual: Scientific Style and Format for Authors, Editors, and Publishers*, Ninth Edition. Council of Science Editors (CSE), University of Chicago Press, 2024.

---

1. Hopkins, A. (2023, January 18). Study Probes Awareness of Alcohol's Link to Cancer. *National Cancer Institute, NIH*. https://www.cancer.gov/news-events/cancer-currents-blog/2023/cancer-alcohol-link-public-awareness

9 | How to Properly Abbreviate a Journal Name

Best Practices

The full names of journals are often abbreviated in the references sections of manuscripts, which reduces the printing costs for the publisher and saves time for authors without access to reference management software. Authors also commonly use journal name abbreviations in grant proposals too. When abbreviating the name of a journal, don't just guess the shortened form. Instead, use an established database to look up the approved journal abbreviation.

The four journal abbreviation databases listed below are the ones most often used within the author guidelines of science journals. If no database is specified in the author guidelines, feel free to use the one you like the best.

- CASSI.[1] The Chemical Abstract Service (CAS), a division of the American Chemical Society, maintains CASSI (CAS Source Index), a comprehensive bibliographic database that contains journal titles, approved abbreviations, and other useful information (e.g., ISBN, ISSN). This database can be searched by using the full journal title or

---

1. Chemical Abstract Service. (n.d.). *CAS Source Index Search Tool*. https://cassi.cas.org/search.jsp

abbreviated name and is quick to use.

- LTWA.[2] The List of Title Word Abbreviations (LTWA) contains all standard title word abbreviations approved by the International Organization for Standardization (ISO). Use the word search tab to look up abbreviations for a word. For example, type in "pharm" to look up the various abbreviations for words containing "pharm" such as pharmacology or pharmacological.
- NLM Catalog.[3] The National Library of Medicine (NLM) Catalog contains bibliographic data on over 1.4 million journals, books, and other resources, including the journals in PubMed. Search this database by using the full journal title; after hitting the search button, select the "Journals currently indexed in MEDLINE" option in the left-hand column to narrow down the search results.
- Index Medicus.[45] This bibliographic database deserves an honorable mention because of its long history dating back to 1879 and its occasional inclusion in journal author instructions. While Index Medicus is limited to journals in biomedicine and is thus not comprehensive, the database can be useful for looking up commonly referenced medical journals, particularly when the abbreviation cannot be located quickly elsewhere. Note, however, that printing of this database ended in 2004 and the content is now a part of MEDLINE, which can be accessed through the NLM Catalog.

Bookmark these databases in a web browser so that each is easy to find.

Lastly, please be aware that if a particular journal's name cannot be found in one of the above databases, journal editors prefer authors include the full title so that in-house staff can choose the appropriate abbreviation. No abbreviation is necessary if the journal's name is a single word.

2. International Standard Serial Number International Centre. (n.d.). *Access to the LTWA*. https://www.issn.org/services/online-services/access-to-the-ltwa/

3. National Library of Medicine. (n.d.). *NLM Catalog*. https://www.ncbi.nlm.nih.gov/nlmcatalog

4. Medical University of Poznań. (n.d.). *Medicus*. http://www.bg.ump.edu.pl/czasopisma/medicus.php?lang=eng

5. *Index Medicus*. (n.d.). In *Wikipedia*. https://en.wikipedia.org/wiki/Index_Medicus

OPTIMIZATION FOR PUBLICATION AND FUNDING

10 | Dos and Don'ts When Writing a Title

> *Key Point*
>
> Good titles for papers or grant proposals are clear, concise, and descriptive.

Best Practices

The title is arguably the most important sentence you will write in a paper or grant proposal. The title is the most widely read part, shapes readers' first impressions, and can influence their decision to read or cite your paper or fund your proposal. Additionally, the title helps people find your content online amongst a mind-boggling amount of competing information. Below is a brief summary of standard advice for writing titles in science.

Dos

- Do write a descriptive title that accurately describes the contents of the paper or proposal.
- Do write a concise title that conforms with any word or character limits.
- Do avoid or minimize acronyms and technical jargon.
- Do use important keywords early on in your title.
- Do realize that several revisions will likely be necessary to achieve an excellent title.

Don'ts

- Don't wait to the last minute to write your title.
- Don't start your title with unnecessary phrases (e.g., Study on) or words (e.g., A, An, The).
- Don't make the title too general.
- Don't use titles that ask questions.
- Don't use funny titles.[1]
- Don't use titles that make declarative statements unless your target journal allows this style.

Further Readings and Resources

- Gastel, B. & Day, R.A. (2022). Chapter 7: How to Prepare the Title. In *How to Write and Publish a Scientific Paper*, Ninth Edition. Greenwood Press, 45–50.
- PLOS Writing Center, How to Write a Great Title. https://plos.org/resource/how-to-write-a-great-title/. The above list structure was adapted from this article.
- Tay, A. (28 July 2020). How to Write a Good Research Paper Title. *Nature News*.

---

1. While these types of titles may work well online in less formal venues, titles used for academic works should have a professional tone.

11 | Use a Formal Tone in Scientific Writing

> *Key Point*
>
> In scientific writing, use a formal tone rather than an informal one because a formal tone helps to convey professionalism and credibility. Key aspects of writing formally include avoiding contractions, slang, and idioms.

Best Practices

Written text can have either a formal or informal tone, but it is best to avoid informal figures of speech when writing grant proposals and manuscripts. Informal expressions are known as colloquialisms (in Latin, colloquor means to converse), and these common components of everyday speech include certain contractions, slang, and idioms.

Contractions are words formed by the omission of a certain letters, such as "didn't" or "can't". These are informal expressions. While it is fine to use a contraction on social media or in a science blog, spell out the contraction in academic papers—for example, did not or cannot.

Slang is informal language particular to a certain group of people. Scientists use many slang terms such as vax for vaccination, lab for laboratory, and DI for deionized water.[1] While it is fine to use such terms over lunch with your labmates, use the full unabbreviated form of the word in your academic papers.

1. Vanity Fair. (2018, March 19). Bill Nye Teaches You Science Slang (video). YouTube. https://www.youtube.com/watch?v=mZq-n3iFr3o

Idioms are phrases that have a meaning that cannot be discerned from the individual words. In the health sciences, popular idioms include "cherry picked," "go viral," "cold feet," and "it's not rocket science." Idioms should be avoided in scientific writing because they are informal and can be difficult to understand for multilingual learners.

Maintaining a formal tone and following other standard writing practices will help ensure that your grant proposals and manuscripts are of the highest quality.

12 | Helpful Tools to Improve the Flow of Logic in Scientific Papers and Proposals

> **Key Point**
>
> Always strive to achieve a clear flow of logic in scientific papers and proposals—this can be accomplished with well-structured outlines, strong topic sentences, parallel constructions, transitional expressions, upfront context statements, and obvious subjects.

Best Practices

Just as a surgeon would not begin a surgery without scalpels, scissors, forceps, and clamps, a scientist should not begin a writing project without knowing how to use a few linguistic tools to optimize the flow of logic. In papers and proposals with clear logic flow, the content can be understood easily and the reader can move effortlessly from sentence to sentence. Any text that causes the reader to pause to comprehend what is being communicated is problematic. Five techniques to optimize the flow of logic, when applied at either the macro level (to the whole paper) or micro level (to words within a sentence), are as follows.

1. **Well-structured outlines.** Construct an outline of the main topics that will be pre-

sented prior to engaging in the writing process—this is a surefire way to achieve a clear flow of logic. Outlines help authors maintain focus and avoid tangents, thereby supporting clarity and conciseness. Hence, invest the time upfront to develop a well-structured outline (or at least a list of bullet points containing the key messages).

2. **Strong topic sentences.** Begin paragraphs with a topic sentence that provides a unifying theme for the sentences that follow. A good topic sentence will improve coherency within the text and serve as a guide for your audience, which consists of busy scientists who often skim through documents. The text below in bold illustrates how the addition of a topic sentence can improve the flow (data are from the National Center for Health Statistics[1]):

   ◦ Without a topic sentence: Heart disease caused 702,880 deaths in the United States in 2022. Cancer caused 608,371 deaths in the United States in 2022. Accidents caused 227,039 deaths in the United States in 2022.
   ◦ With a topic sentence: **The leading causes of death in the United States in 2022 were heart disease, cancer, and accidents.** Heart disease caused 702,880 deaths, cancer caused 608,371 deaths, and accidents caused 227,039 deaths.

3. **Parallel constructions.** Use the same grammatical structure in headers, specific aims statements, paragraphs, sentences, tables, and figures because parallelism is critical to achieving a clear flow of logic. These phrasings have a parallel structure: identify, determine, assess; these phrasings do not: identify, determination, assessing. Similarly, if the topic sentence states that you collected data during week 1, week 4, and week 12, discuss the data in that order to maintain a parallel structure. Parallel constructions facilitate understanding in a profound way. This will be one of the sharpest tools in your toolbox.

4. **Transitional expressions.** Let the reader know what to expect with transitional expressions. Common ones used in scientific papers include however, additionally, furthermore, importantly, subsequently, consequently, therefore, hence, thus, and finally. More examples can be found in the logical relationship–transitional expression table created by the Writing Center at University of North Carolina at Chapel Hill.[2]

5. **Upfront context statements.** Move ending phrases that give temporal or spatial con-

1. Center for Disease Control and Prevention. (2024, May 2). *Leading Causes of Death*. National Center for Health Statistics. https://www.cdc.gov/nchs/fastats/leading-causes-of-death.htm

text to a sentence, such as "in earlier experiments" and "in several patients," to the first part of a sentence. Readers will then immediately understand the context for the information that comes next.

6. **Obvious subjects.** Scrutinize the use of "it" and "this/these" for brevity. Often the use of such terms is entirely appropriate, but be sure that readers will not need to waste precious time figuring out the correct subject. This can occur if "it" or "this/these" could refer to more than one noun in the preceding text. Simply replacing the words "it" and "this/these" with more specific terminology in such situations can prevent any misunderstanding.

2. University of North Carolina at Chapel Hill. (n.d). *Transitions*. The Writing Center. https://writingcenter.unc.edu/tips-and-tools/transitions/

13 | Ways to Minimize Jargon

> *Key Point*
>
> Minimize the use of jargon to produce clear and concise scientific documents.

Best Practices

The online Merriam-Webster dictionary defines jargon as (1) "technical terminology or characteristic idiom of a special activity or group" and (2) "obscure and often pretentious language marked by circumlocutions and long words."[1] Jargon can make a paper or proposal difficult to read and unnecessarily long. Thankfully, there are easy ways to minimize jargon.

First, identify all technical terms in the writing that readers from a variety of backgrounds may not readily understand. Then, define those terms when introduced.

Another easy way to minimize jargon is to replace problematic phrases with less wordy alternatives. Lists can be helpful for this purpose. Below is a sample list that can be built upon, and it would be well worth the time and effort to develop a personalized list that is more comprehensive.

Lengthy and obtuse phrases followed by suggested substitutes:[2]

---

1. Merriam-Webster. (n.d.). Jargon. In *Merriam-Webster.com dictionary*. https://www.merriam-webster.com/dictionary/jargon

2. Adapted from Appendix 2: Words and Expressions to Avoid in *How to Write and Publish a Scientific Paper*, Ninth Edition. Greenwood Press, 2022, 348.

Jargon	Substitute
A large number of	Many
Anti-cancer therapeutic	Cancer treatment
At an earlier point in time	Previously
Despite the fact that	Although
During the course of	During, while
In order to	To
It is important to note	Importantly
On a daily basis	Daily
Post surgery	After surgery
Tumored	Injected with tumor cells
Utilization	Use
We wish to thank	We thank

Some authors might find it easiest to just write what comes naturally and then edit the text to reduce jargon. However, over time, use of clear and concise terminology will become a habit during the writing process.

14 | Don't Bury the Lede of a Grant Proposal

Key Point

Summarize the most important and intriguing aspects of a grant proposal in the introductory paragraph to grab the reviewers' attention.

Best Practices

Journalists frequently repeat the adage "don't bury the lede," and this advice works well for grant proposals too. The lede[1] refers to the opening lines of a story that give the reader a preview of what is to come. When someone buries the lede, they position the most important parts of the story well beneath other minor details. Start paying closer attention to the ledes in science news stories online and what constitutes a good lede will become clear.

Does the lede give the gist of the who, what, where, when, why, and how? Does the lede create curiosity and a desire to keep reading? If yes, then the author wrote a good lede.

A well-structured lede about an important problem aligned with the research priorities of a funding announcement or review panel can be a huge asset in the Specific Aims section of a National Institutes of Health (NIH) grant proposal. In particular, such a lede can compel busy reviewers, who often have to read dozens of proposals, to delve into your proposal

1. The spelling of lede is thought to have originated in newsrooms in the 1970s, where the play on words helped people distinguish between story ledes and the metal leads in Linotype machines separating the lines of type. Merriam-Webster added lede to the dictionary in 2008. Merriam-Webster. (n.d.). *Why do we 'bury the lede?'* https://www.merriam-webster.com/wordplay/bury-the-lede-versus-lead

more closely. Additionally, it may even help them to recall your proposal more readily during the latter parts of the review process.

Scientists struggle to write good ledes because that is not how they have been trained to write. In a scientific paper, the motivations for the research and the logical arguments underpinning the interpretations of the results are divulged little by little as build-up to a grand conclusion—the very antithesis of using a lede. To start writing ledes for grant proposals, it may help to focus on what makes the research impactful and highlight that upfront. For example, does the research have the potential to improve survival outcomes in patients with hard-to-treat cancers, or will it help doctors to personalize treatments so that the most effective ones can be used? Stating such long-term goals upfront will make the proposal more attractive to funders, who may miss these important impact statements when they are positioned lower in a proposal.

Below are examples of effective ledes drawn respectively from a news story and a successful grant proposal:

> *The World Health Organization (WHO) is taking on the world's worst killer, laying out its first plan to conquer hypertension—a level of high blood pressure that affects one in every three adults globally. That figure has doubled since 1990. It's now up to 1.3 billion people.*[2]

> *Over the past two decades, excess dietary intake and low physical activity have contributed to an increase in the prevalence of childhood obesity in the United States, affecting a third of children and disproportionately impacting minority and economically disadvantaged children. Given that obesity is a risk factor for health outcomes later in life, including cancer, early obesity prevention efforts are critical for population health.*[3]

Like all things, writing good ledes for your grant proposals will become easier with practice.

---

2. Maryn, M. (2023, September 19). High Blood Pressure Is The World's Biggest Killer. Now There's a Plan to Tackle It. *Wired*. https://www.wired.com/story/high-blood-pressure-is-the-worlds-biggest-killer-now-theres-a-plan-to-tackle-it/

3. Rebekka Mairghread Lee, ScD, Harvard School of Public Health, R21: Effective Training Models for Implementing Health-Promoting Practices Afterschool, https://cancercontrol.cancer.gov/sites/default/files/2020-05/SGA_9182511.pdf. Sample proposal via the National Cancer Institute (NCI) at https://cancercontrol.cancer.gov/is/funding/sample-grant-applications.

15 | Four Search Engine Optimization Tools to Boost a Paper's Citation Rate

Key Point

Using search engine optimization strategies before and after publication of an academic paper can increase the number of people who view, read, and cite it.

Best Practices

Search engine optimization (SEO) is a process for helping a webpage appear closer to the top in a list of search engine results, which can drive more traffic to the content. When computer bots crawl over a paper's abstract on PubMed or the journal's table of contents, they will look for things like keywords and backlinks from your institutional biography page. Using the four strategies described below will help to ensure that a paper's abstract is indexed properly (i.e., how the data are categorized and stored by a search engine) and ranked highly in search engines like Google, Google Scholar, and Bing.

1. **Choose good keywords.** Start by selecting three to four suitable keywords or keyword phrases for your research, along the lines of what an interested reader may use to search for similar content in PubMed. Then, test those keywords in a keyword finder/planner (e.g., Google Ads Keyword Plan tool, Wordtracker, which can be accessed by signing up for an online account)—these planners show the number of times a particular phrase and its synonyms have been searched for over a set timeframe. Lastly, use

this information to optimize the paper's keywords. Ideally, those keywords should correspond to the most popular, relevant terms being used during internet searches, which will improve the paper's rank in search engine results.

2. **Write a search-friendly title.** Include your most important keyword in the first 60 characters of the title. Computer bots are programmed for speed and search only the first 60 or so characters of titles. If the first portion of a title lacks this keyword, the bots may give it short shrift. Because title keywords are weighted heavily during the crawling, indexing, and ranking processes, you want the most important one to count.

3. **Reword the abstract.** Repeat your most important keyword 3–4 times in the abstract, and use the other keywords in the first two sentences, i.e., content that the bots will focus on. Repetition of keywords teaches the bots that these phrases are important. However, don't stuff the abstract full of keywords. Attempts to cheat the system in this way can actually hurt a paper's SEO ranking.

4. **Build links.** Link to the paper's abstract from your institutional biography page and social media accounts (e.g., LinkedIn). As the bots crawl over the paper's abstract and discover backlinks, these signal that the content is credible and thus deserves a higher rank.

The above SEO strategies will make your paper easier to discover online and may even boost its citation rate and impact.

THE PUBLICATION PROCESS

16 | Journal Selection Simplified

Key Point

Selection of an appropriate science journal for a manuscript is an important part of the publication process and should be carried out in a thoughtful manner.

Best Practices

Too often researchers rush through the journal selection process and pick a target journal that is not a good venue for their unpublished paper. Inevitably, this haste results in numerous rejections and an inefficient use of time for both authors and journal editors. Yes, the journal selection process is not always easy, but it is well worth the effort to do it well. In particular, selection of a journal that is a good fit for a manuscript can boost readership numbers and save valuable time during the publication process. Below are some factors to consider during the journal selection process and three steps to make this complex process more manageable.

First and foremost, the paper needs to fit well with the scope of the journal and be well matched in terms of the journal's prestige and readership base. Use a reasonable range of competitiveness (from conservative to aspirational) based on the significance of the findings, and think through who will be most likely to read the paper. Besides scope fit, impact, and intended audience, there are a whole host of other factors to consider, such as fees, open access policies, acceptance rates, and publication frequency.

Try the following three steps as a decision-support tool (feel free to modify the content below to best suit your needs). Doing so may not only lead to a better decision, but also impress your co-authors with your thoroughness.

1. Develop a starter list of 5–10 potential journals.

   a. Run a keyword search in reference databases, such as Scopus, Web of Science, PubMed, and Google Scholar. Take note of the journals that appear on the first two or three pages of results for both the newest papers and the most relevant papers.

   b. Review the reference list (if completed) or collection of papers that will be cited. Take note of any journals for papers that are foundational to your research. Whenever possible, it is a good practice to cite at least one paper from the target journal, which helps to demonstrate the good scope fit.

   c. Ask a co-author or mentor if they have suggestions.

   d. If you are a member of a scientific society that publishes a journal, consider adding that one to the starter list if it is not yet on it.

2. Narrow down the list to the top three journals for further consideration.

   a. Collect comprehensive data on your top three choices (journal name, website link, Editor-in-Chief, journal impact factor, brief scope description, publication frequency, publication fees, open access options, turn-around times, acceptance rate, size restrictions, formatting-free submissions, years in existence). It may be helpful to organize these data in a table. Note that you may not be able to fill in all of the data points for some journals, as journals do not always make that information available online.

   b. If at any time you find that a journal being researched in depth is not suitable for your paper (paper greatly exceeds the size limit requirements, publication fees are too high), simply delete that choice and move on to another journal you identified in step 1.

3. Rank the top three journals, and submit your paper to your top choice. If that journal rejects your paper, consider the next one down in this prioritized list as well as any others recommended by the journal editors.

Whenever possible, select the target journal before drafting the paper. That way the content can be geared toward the journal's scope and formatted properly at the outset.

Authors might also find it useful to explore online journal finders to support their decision-making.[1]

1. This content would be useful for a training exercise in which participants are asked to select two or three suitable journals for a paper.

17 | Don't Fall Prey to Predatory Journals

Key Point

Verify that the target journal is not a predatory journal prior to submitting a paper for publication.

Best Practices

The number of scientific journals has grown explosively in recent years, but not all journals are suitable venues for academic research. Nowadays, care is needed to ensure that a target journal is not a predatory one. In simplest terms, a predatory journal is one that engages in unethical publishing practices. Reputable journals routinely perform services like peer review, copy editing, abstracting and indexing, paper archiving, errata postings, and managing conflicts of interest. These services are supported by subscription fees or open access fees obtained from authors. Some reputable journals will even help to promote the research they publish on social media. In contrast, predatory publishers are profit-motivated entities that often skip or scrimp on such steps to keep costs low, which leads to the publication of poor-quality papers and shoddy science. A few predatory journals have even fabricated their editorial boards and faked journal impact factors. Steer clear of them. If a paper is inadvertently published in a predatory journal, at best it will be ignored by the scientific community, but at worst, it could hurt the author's credibility.

Unfortunately, there is currently no systematic way to identify predatory journals with ease. Several lists of questionable journals have popped up over the years, but use of such lists can be problematic. Specifically, these lists can mistakenly omit a predatory journal if the list is not updated regularly, or these lists can erroneously identify a small, under-resourced journal as predatory when in reality it is not. My best advice to avoid predatory journals is to be aware of the problem, use established databases to look up reputable publishers (Directory of Open Access Journals (DOAJ), ISSN Portal, Ulrichsweb Global Serials Directory), verify journal impact factors, and know the warning signs. Consultation with a medical librarian also can be incredibly helpful.[1]

The National Institutes of Health (NOT-OD-18-011) offers these characteristics of disreputable publishers:[2]

- *misleading pricing (e.g., lack of transparency about article processing charges);*
- *failure to disclose information to authors;*
- *aggressive tactics to solicit article submissions;*
- *inaccurate statements about editorial board membership; and*
- *misleading or suspicious peer-review processes.*

For example, predatory journals may not disclose their office location and often send multiple emails to authors to urge a submission.

Be on the lookout for inaccessible or odd-looking contact information, poorly designed websites, unrealistic peer-review and publication timelines, or reluctance to turn over copyright despite fees paid for fully open access articles. Reach out to the members of the editorial board if you have questions about their involvement.

A powerful system that has been developed by the scholarly publishing community is "Think. Check. Submit."[3] Think: is this a trusted journal; Check: assess the journal with the checklist below; Submit: only submit your paper to a journal that has been verified to be a reputable source.

1. Gastel (2021). Choosing a Journal for Submission: Don't Fall Prey. *Methodist Debakey Cardiovascular Journal*, 17(4), 90–92. https://doi.org/10.14797/mdevj.650.

2. National Institutes of Health. (2017, November 3). *Statement on Article Publication Resulting from NIH Funded Research.* https://grants.nih.gov/grants/guide/notice-files/NOT-OD-18-011.html

3. Think. Check. Submit. (n.d). https://thinkchecksubmit.org/

Journal checklist to assess if a journal is trusted from Think. Check. Submit. (This content, duplicated here, is licensed under a Creative Commons Attribution 4.0 International License.[4])

Do you or your colleagues know the journal?

- Have you read any articles in the journal before?
- Is it easy to discover the latest papers in the journal?
- Name of the journal: the name is unique; it is not the same or easily confused with another journal.
- Can you cross check with information about the journal in the ISSN portal?

Can you easily identify and contact the publisher?

- Is the publisher name clearly displayed on the journal website?
- Can you contact the publisher by telephone, email, and post?

Is the journal clear about the type of peer review it uses?

- Does the website mention whether the process involves independent/external reviewers, how many reviewers per paper?
- Is the publisher offering a review by an expert editorial board or by researchers in your subject area?
- The journal doesn't guarantee acceptance or a very short peer review time.

Are articles indexed and/or archived in dedicated services?

- Will your work be indexed/archived in an easily discoverable database?
- Does the publisher ensure long term archiving and preservation of digital publications?
- Does the publisher use permanent digital identifiers?

Is it clear what fees will be charged?

- Does the journal site explain what these fees are for and when they will be charged?
- Does the publisher explain on their website how they are financially supported?
- Do they mention the currency and amount of any fees?
- Does the publisher website explain whether or not waivers are available?

Are guidelines provided for authors on the publisher website?

- For open access journals, does the publisher have a clear license policy? Are there preferred licenses? Are there exceptions permitted depending on the needs of the author? Are license details included on all publications?
- Does the publisher allow you to retain copyright of your work? Can you share your work via, for example, an institutional repository, and under what terms?
- Does the publisher have a clear policy regarding potential conflicts of interest for authors, editors, and reviewers?
- Can you tell what formats your paper will be available in? (e.g. HTML, XML, PDF)
- Does the journal provide any information about metrics of usage or citations?

4. Think. Check. Submit. (n.d.). *Journals.* https://thinkchecksubmit.org/journals/

Is the publisher a current member of a recognized industry initiative?

- Are they a current member of the Committee on Publication Ethics (COPE) and follow its guidelines?
- If the journal is open access, is it listed in the Directory of Open Access Journals (DOAJ)?
- If the publisher offers an open access option, is it a current member of the Open Access Scholarly Publishers' Association (OASPA)?
- Is the journal hosted on one of INASP's Journals Online platforms (for journals published in Bangladesh, Nepal, Sri Lanka, Central America, and Mongolia) or on African Journals Online (AJOL, for African journals)?
- If the journal is open access, is it hosted on Scielo (for Latin American scientific journals)?
- If the journal is open access, is it indexed in Latindex (for journals that are published in Latin America, the Caribbean, Spain, and Portugal)?
- If the journal is open access, is it indexed by Redalyc (for journals that are published in Latin America and the Caribbean, Spain, and Portugal)?
- Is the publisher a member of another trade association?

18 | Beware of Zombie Papers

Key Point

Thoroughly check manuscripts just prior to publication to ensure that a retracted paper has not been cited inappropriately.

Best Practices

Here's a scary scenario: a journal editor issues a warning about your recently published paper because a retracted paper was inadvertently cited without noting the retraction. Papers that have been retracted but continue to be cited in the literature as valid work are known as zombie papers, and citations to zombie papers are frighteningly routine.[1] Even scarier are the possibilities that your paper could get tagged with an expression of concern from a journal editor for a wrongful citation or that someone could make medical decisions hinging on the flawed science. Hence, take care to avoid citing a zombie paper.

First, know that not all journals screen reference lists within papers in press for retracted paper citations. Thus, even though this practice is becoming more commonplace among publishers thanks to a recommendation issued by the International Committee of Medical Journal Editors (ICMJE), do not rely on a journal-initiated screen to protect the integrity of your paper. Instead, you or an associate should cross-check each reference cited in a paper against the online abstract at the publisher's website where retraction notices are posted. It's

---

1. Content was originally used in a Roswell Park newsletter distributed on Halloween. Further distribution around the time of this holiday is encouraged.

important to use the publisher's website because retractions are not always noted in popular databases like Google Scholar. While recent retraction notices can be found reliably in PubMed, use caution with older papers.

Second, if you do find a retracted paper in your preprint's references section, don't panic. Carefully consider whether excluding this paper will alter the conclusions. If not, simply remove it from the references. However, if the paper helped to inform the research in a substantial way, you will need to redo the analyses and possibly even some of the experiments. This prospect may make your blood run cold, but it is the responsible thing to do.

Third, if a reference to a retracted paper must be included, cite the retraction notice and not the original paper. Explanatory text will likely be needed to justify the decision to use this strategy. One possible reason to cite a retracted paper is when the uncertainty created in the wake of the retraction needs to be discussed directly.[2]

The above steps will help you to steer clear of any scientific horror stories. Share this new-found knowledge about zombie papers with colleagues. We can all help to fight this scourge.

2. Committee on Publication Ethics. (2015). *Citing a retracted paper.* https://publicationethics.org/case/citing-retracted-paper

19 | How to Respond to Reviewers' Comments

Best Practices

Even the best manuscripts and grant proposals will receive some unfavorable comments during the peer-review process, so don't be disheartened. Instead, take time to cool down and reflect on the comments. You will then be better prepared to respond appropriately. In the written response,

1. **Be organized.** Start with an introductory statement in which the reviewers are thanked for their involvement and summarize the major changes that were made to the paper or proposal. Then, address the comments systematically. For manuscripts, each comment should be copied exactly as it was provided, and your response should follow. Often it helps to use a different formatting style (e.g., color) to distinguish the reviewers' comments from the responses. Your individual responses should begin with a clear and concise statement describing the overall response (agreed, changed as requested, unable to address because this was beyond the scope of the study); next, detail the changes that were made and either copy the newly revised text into this document with block quotes (indented and italicized text) or provide the exact page and line numbers where the reviewers can examine the tracked changes that were made. For

grant proposals, in which your response may be restricted to one page, group the reviewers' concerns into similar themes and respond topically (under the headings Significance, Investigator, Innovation, Approach, Environment). A common error is to ignore or incompletely address some comments—this will hurt your chances of emerging successfully from peer review.

2. **Be professional.** Always use courteous language and respond in a diplomatic and timely manner. Passionate defenses of the research will not work in your favor. Maintain a professional and objective tone even if the reviewers did not.

3. **Be constructive.** In general, accommodate all of the requested changes that are easy to address and improve the content. For requested changes that are more difficult to implement, do your best to understand why this issue was flagged during peer review and identify workable solutions; then, clearly explain how the changes are responsive to this comment within the limits of what is possible. Lastly, if you disagree with the requested change, politely state why and fully justify your decision. In preparing your responses, it will help to adopt the perspective of reviewers who must evaluate whether the changes or lack thereof are acceptable.

In conclusion, one word can summarize how best to respond to reviewers' comments: carefully!

Further Readings and Resources

- Curran-Everett, D. (2017). The thrill of the paper, the agony of the review. *Advances in Physiology Education*, 41, 338–340. https://doi.org/10.1152/advan.00069.2017
- Nahata, M.C. & Sorkin, E.M. (2019). Responding to manuscript reviewer and editor comments. *Annals of Pharmacotherapy*, 53(9), 959–961. https://doi.org/10.1177/1060028019849941
- Noble, W.S. (2017). Ten simple rules for writing a response to reviewers. *PLoS Computational Biology*, 13(10), article no. e1005730. https://doi.org/10.1371/journal.pcbi.1005730

20 | How to Give Good Feedback on Colleagues' Drafts

Key Point

Always strive to give respectful, actionable, and prioritized feedback when peer reviewing colleagues' academic writing projects.[1]

Best Practices

When a colleague asks for a review of their manuscript or grant proposal, they likely view you as a trusted source of wisdom. Embrace this opportunity for collaboration—as a subject matter expert in the field or not, you have value to offer as a reader of an early or later draft. Is the content clear? Is the logic sound? What is the most compelling aspect of this work? Authors are often too engrossed in the details to grasp higher-level perspectives that can turn a decent piece of writing into an extraordinary one. To help them along, use the mnemonic device RAP (Respectful, Actionable, Prioritized): the corresponding advice will help you to avoid a bad "RAP" from a few botched reviews and learn to give constructive feedback that is important for building a good RAPport with colleagues.

---

1. This material was adapted from the following article: Botham, C.M., Brawn, S., Steele, L., Barrón, C.B., Kleppner, S.R., & Herschlag, D. (2020). Biosciences Proposal Bootcamp: Structured peer and faculty feedback improves trainees' proposals and grantsmanship self-efficacy. *PLoS ONE*, 15(12), article no. e0243973. https://doi.org/10.1371/journal.pone.0243973

1. **Respectful comments.** There are many aspects of giving respectful feedback. For starters, choose words carefully when adding critical comments to a document. Authors will be more receptive to comments if they are phrased as suggestions or questions versus mandates. Second, be timely with feedback (it is always best to give an author plenty of time to review and act on your comments). Third, remark on both the strengths of the writing as well as its weaknesses. Lastly, withhold judgment on a poorly written first draft because the final version may turn out to be phenomenal. In that situation, a good strategy is to provide high-level comments about topics, like what's missing and what needs more attention, and offer to provide more detailed comments or revisions in a later draft.

2. **Actionable advice.** When commenting, avoid ambiguous statements like "the meaning in this paragraph is not clear"; instead query, do you mean this or that and point out what specific wording is problematic. Additionally, don't recommend actions that are not feasible. For example, if a document has already been through a pre-submission inquiry or the peer-review process, the author may not be able to rewrite whole sections. Also, be aware that lengthy new experiments may not be possible if there is a tight publishing timeline or budget. A good practice is to inquire with the author about what types of feedback they want.

3. **Prioritized recommendations.** Last but not least, prioritize! Shape the feedback according to the author's stated needs and timeframe for the review. Try not to give too much feedback or you risk overwhelming the author and using your time inefficiently; conversely, try not to give too little feedback if improvements are warranted because help is clearly wanted. Importantly, focus time and effort on the highest points of leverage for improving the document. Your role in this is as a peer reviewer of a colleague's work and not that of an editor or publisher with the responsibility for eliminating all errors.

Again, the mnemonic device RAP (Respectful, Actionable, Prioritized) can help with remembering these tips. Giving good feedback is important for building a good rapport with colleagues and promoting their success.

LIVE AUDIENCES

21 | Tips for Delivering Effective Presentations

> *Key Point*
>
> Maintain an audience-focused mindset to help create powerful presentations.

Best Practices

Many of us begin planning a presentation by asking ourselves what we want to say and how best to organize that information. In practice, however, broadening your mindset to include both what you want to say and what your audience will find the most helpful to hear can be instrumental for delivering highly effective presentations. Below are a few tips that may help.[1]

1. **Minimize jargon.** Are you presenting to your lab group where everyone is well acquainted with the research topic, or are you presenting to a larger group of scientists at a departmental seminar or conference where people have only a broad understanding of the research topic? Perhaps there are members of the news media or patient advocates in your audience. Knowing your audience can help you to gauge how many technical terms and acronyms are reasonable to use. In general, minimize use of highly technical terminology to promote broad understanding of the topic.

2. **Provide context.** Take time upfront to explain why the topic is important to you and

---

1. *Attribution note:* These tips were shared with the author during a science communication training session with the Alan Alda Center for Communicating Science, hosted by the Society of Toxicology on October 28, 2022. Further dissemination of the communication tips was a condition of the training award.

your audience. While all audience members will benefit from some sort of framing, certain people will clearly require more background information at the outset than others to truly understand what is being communicated. If instead you dive right into the details of the scientific research, you risk losing their attention.

3. **Use large font sizes.** Nothing is worse than settling in to enjoy a presentation and being barely able to read the slides. Hence, make sure the content is readable from a reasonable distance, and don't cram too much information on any one slide. The Association of Research Libraries recommends a minimum font size of 24 points.[2]

4. **Focus on a limited number of essential messages.** You will be lucky if your audience can recall more than one or two key points after some time has passed following the presentation. Thus, distill down the information you want to present, and keep the key points simple and easy to remember. The essential messages should be of value to your audience in some way. Repeat your most important messages more than once, such as in the results and summary.

5. **Stay within the time limit.** Any information presented in rush mode will not be retained well. Therefore, it is critical to time your talk beforehand and trim the content down if necessary. Leave time for questions.

6. **Engage the audience.** Audiences largely do not like it when presenters read directly from their presentation notes. A better strategy is to create bullets of your talking points as a guide and memorize only the transitions; then, discuss the content in a clear, conversational manner. Alternatively, if the presentation is very important and you have ample time to practice, you can memorize the presentation (though practice enough to not sound stilted and lose your place if there are interruptions). In terms of delivery, it is important to make eye contact often and use hand gestures to convey enthusiasm.

The adage "know your audience" is crucial for delivering effective presentations. If you are not following the above tips already, test them out for your next talk—your audience will thank you for it.

2. Association of Research Libraries. (n.d.). *PowerPoint guidelines for Presenters*. https://www.arl.org/accessibility-guidelines-for-power-point-presentations/

Recommended Further Readings and Resources

AMA Manual of Style: A Guide for Authors and Editors, 11th Edition. American Medical Association (AMA), Oxford University Press, 2020.

AuthorAID. https://www.authoraid.info/en/

Barnard, S.R. & St. James, D. *Listen. Write. Present. The Elements for Communicating Science and Technology.* New Haven and London: Yale University Press, 2012.

CLIMB (Collaborative Learning and Integrated Mentoring in the Biosciences). Creating Coherent Paragraphs: Topic Sentences, Echo Words, Transitions. Northwestern University. Retrieved on July 12, 2024, https://www.northwestern.edu/climb/resources/written-communication/Creating-Coherent-Paragraphs.html

Clinical Chemistry Guide to Scientific Writing. Clinical Chemistry, Oxford Academic. https://academic.oup.com/clinchem/pages/guide-to-scientific-writing

Flanagin, A., Frey, T., & Christiansen, M.A. (2021). Updated Guidance on the Reporting of Race and Ethnicity in Medical and Science Journals. *JAMA*, 326(7), 621–627. https://jamanetwork.com/journals/jama/fullarticle/2783090

Gastel, B. & Day, R.A. *How to Write and Publish a Scientific Paper*, Ninth Edition. Greenwood Press, 2022.

Gopen, G. & Swan, J. (2018). The Science of Scientific Writing. *American Scientist*, 78(6), 550–558.

Matthews, J.R. & Matthews, R.W. *Successful Scientific Writing: A Step-by-Step Guide for the Biological and Medical Sciences*, Fourth Edition. Cambridge, UK: Cambridge University Press, 2014.

National Institute of Allergy and Infectious Diseases (NIAID). Apply for a Grant [website]. National Institutes of Health. https://www.niaid.nih.gov/grants-contracts/apply-grant

Pinker, S. *The Sense of Style: The Thinking Person's Guide to Writing in the 21st Century*. New York, NY: Penguin, 2014.

Publication Manual of the American Psychological Association, Seventh Edition. American Psychological Association (APA), 2019.

Purdue OWL: Online Writing Lab (OWL), Purdue University, https://owl.purdue.edu/.

Recommendations for the Conduct, Reporting, Editing, and Publication of Scholarly Work in Medical Journals. International Committee of Medical Journal Editors (ICMJE), 2024.

Robertson, J.D., Russell, S.W., & Morrison, D.C. The Grant Application Writer's Workbook: National Institutes of Health Version. Grant Writer's Seminars and Workshops (GWSW), 2024.

Sakaduski, N. & Day, R.A. *Scientific English: A Guide for Scientists and Other Professionals*. Greenwood, 2011.

Strohmeier, A., Plain Language for Researchers. Clinical and Translational Science Institute, University at Buffalo. Retrieved on July 11, 2024 from https://www.buffalo.edu/ctsi/cores/clinical-research-office/educational-modules/plain-language-for-researchers.html

Strunk, W., Jr. & White, E.B. *The Elements of Style*, Fiftieth Anniversary Edition. New York: Pearson Longman, 2008.

The Chicago Manual of Style, 18th Edition. University of Chicago Press, 2024.

The CSE Manual: Scientific Style and Format for Authors, Editors, and Publishers, Ninth Edition. Council of Science Editors (CSE), University of Chicago Press, 2024.

The Writing Center, University of North Carolina at Chapel Hill. https://writingcenter.unc.edu/

University Writing Center, Texas A&M University. https://writingcenter.tamu.edu/

Zeiger, M. *Essentials of Writing Biomedical Research Papers*, Second Edition. McGraw Hill, 1999.

Zinsser, W. *On Writing Well: The Classic Guide to Writing Nonfiction*. Harper Collins, 2016.

Acknowledgments

The author thanks Dr. Sandra O. Gollnick, Professor Emeritus, Roswell Park Comprehensive Cancer Center, for help with selecting the topics to write about and critical reviews of the editorial advice for accuracy and clarity. Thanks are also owed to various other colleagues at Roswell Park who occasionally contributed suggestions to write about and provided insights into the potential uses of this content. Ms. Judith G. Epstein helped proofread the final version.

The author is grateful to the external peer reviewers, Dr. Joanna Downer, Associate Dean for Research Development, Duke University School of Medicine, and Dr. Barbara Gastel, Professor, Texas A&M University, for their constructive reviews of this e-book.

Lastly, the author thanks Ms. Allison Brown, Digital Publishing Services Manager, Charlie Wilson, and others at Milne Open Textbooks, State University of New York (SUNY) at Geneseo, for their assistance with navigating the publication process and assembling the final product.

The Scientific Editing and Research Communications Core (SERCC) is an institutionally funded shared resource that receives support from Roswell Park Comprehensive Cancer Center and National Cancer Institute grant P30CA016056, as well as the Roswell Park Alliance Foundation.

About the Author

Deanna Erin Conners, MS, PhD

Deanna Erin Conners is a senior scientific editor and director of the editing shared resource at Roswell Park Comprehensive Cancer Center in Buffalo, New York. She holds a PhD in Toxicology and has more than 12 years of experience in the field of scientific communication. Dr. Conners has edited more than 2,000 projects in diverse fields for academic scientists and is well acquainted with the needs of early career faculty and multilingual authors.

Made in the USA
Columbia, SC
13 April 2025

56555789R00043